BRAIN HEALTH PROTOCOL

An Alzheimer's Defense

By Steven James Sargent

Preface

The brain is the most complex organ in the body. Any number of conditions can attack and damage the brain. In 2010 my dad died of Alzheimer's. That's when my journey began. I really didn't know much about this debilitating disease but I knew that I did not want his fate to be my fate. To that end I started studying possible causes and preventative measures. I looked at clinical studies, herbal medicine, and ancient remedies. I was willing to consider anything short of incantations and witchcraft.

I discovered early in my quest that I was already doing some of the things that were considered preventative measures: weight training; cutting out sugars; and eating foods that would reduce inflammation in the body,-- including the brain-- but I was sure there had to be more that I could do.

The fact that two of my dad's six sisters had also been diagnosed with AD, gave me additional motivation. And then I began to get news of more people I knew with the disease -- my first drum instructor, Ed

Hamrick, and the father of my friend Brian along with several others. I don't know if my newfound awareness of AD brought these cases more into focus or if was happening more frequently across the board. As it turns out, from my research I found that AD is becoming more frequent.

Although the increase in documented cases of Alzheimer's in recent years may be to some degree attributed to improved reporting methods, the fact remains that medical science recognizes that of those individuals who live to age 85, 1 in 3 will be diagnosed with Alzheimer's or some form of dementia.

Alzheimer's is currently the 7th leading cause of death in the US and is the most common cause of dementia. Almost 6.5 million Americans are living currently living with AD. That's an increase of 700,000 in just three years. That number is expected to exceed 13 million by 2060. AD doesn't only change the life of the patient. More than 11 million family members and unpaid caregivers were affected in 2019.

What's particularly disturbing is that the average age of dementia and AD patients is getting younger. It's becoming more common with people in their 40s and occurs as early as the 20s. This is no longer a disease that we may have to deal with only in our later years.

If you are reading this, you have likely already read many publications and studies and found, as I have, that there is more ambiguity than answers. We find most studies chocked with subjective terms such as "could be," "may be," "and "possibly." Those are not words we want to hear when we're searching for life-or-death answers, particularly when we know it will be a slow death. When medical science tells you that there is no cure for Alzheimer's what they are actually saying is there is not a cure within their pharmaceutical parameters. Furthermore, before a treatment can be declared a cure, it would have to be approved by the FDA in America or other government agencies internationally and natural remedies can't be patented and they are simply not profitable.

Before we get deep into the weeds of natural remedies, I want to direct you to a few articles online that might help to clarify some misconceptions regarding modern medicine.

Rather than offering you a link, I will suggest using search terms.

Go to potency710.com and search "How John D Rockefeller influenced modern medicine."

Veriheal.com
"Rockefellers influence on modern medicine."

Meridianhealthclinic.com
"how Rockefeller created the business of modern medicine."

Chapter 1: The Causes

For many years amyloid plaques were a primary suspect in AD and dementia. More recent studies have shown that hypothesis to be false. Research has discovered that amyloid plaques are a consequence of AD, not a cause. The scientific method itself may indicate the reason the cure has not yet been found. Scientists look at a possibility and spend decades determining whether or not this possibility is the culprit. Many years pass before medical researchers move on to find another possibility.

Science moves slowly and takes time. The person who has been diagnosed with AD does not have time. Time is the enemy. That person needs answers as soon as possible.

I am not a doctor. Like you, I am a consumer of health care. I don't consider myself an expert in this field but instead, a librarian who knows where to access the information.

I started in 1985 with an obsession for nutrition and fitness which gave me a baseline from which to work. At the time, most of my study came from muscle magazines, which contain a great deal of information with regard to proper nutrition, herbs, and other supplements that optimize health, not just for bodybuilding, but for good health in general.

When my Dad was diagnosed, it was like a slap in the face. I didn't know anything about AD or any other brain ailment. I had been told that heredity was a factor and that's all I needed to know. So, I had work to do.

I decided to develop a warrior mindset in the prevention of AD. I looked at every possibility that I could find on the internet and traced back exactly why each possible remedy might work. I looked at origins, history, case studies, control group testing, anecdotal evidence, and whatever was available. I did not discount anything.

In the past decade, some of what I learned early on fell flat, some had moderate success and some remedies have passed greater scrutiny. Those that I believe to be beneficial and from sources I have found to be reliable over time and are remedies that I subscribe to in my daily regimen. Those are included in the following pages. Much of what you will find in this guide will prove to be beneficial in the treatment of other conditions that you may suffer from.

Much of what I will suggest in this book may seem completely foreign to you. Much of it may seem over the top. Much of the nutrition information herein may run counter to doctors' recommendations and TV commercials that tell you how healthy certain foods are.

On average, Doctors spent an average of 19.5 hours of their academic career studying nutrition and are now too busy working to keep up with the most recent nutritional studies. The purveyors of your favorite breakfast cereal have a product to sell and the corporate bottom line is the objective, not the health of their customers. Yet, advertisers have for years tagged foods with little or no positive nutritional value with terms like "part of a balanced diet" or "heart healthy." We have been conditioned to believe these terms.

https://youtu.be/sVISEWacOa

Search for; theatlantic.com
"Why cereal has such aggressive marketing."

Chapter 2: Know Your Enemy

Let's begin by arming you with knowledge. In this chapter, we will dispel some untruths and help you develop some new habits that will put you on the right track. Keep in mind that by simply taking on new routines and changing your daily modus operandi, you are exercising your brain. That being the case, embrace the change.

These are the factors we will cover:

- **Genetics is a factor however,** having the genes that are common markers of AD doesn't mean you are doomed.
- **What we think we know.** Watch the YouTube video on

the channel named " Scishow"
titled "We might be totally wrong
about Alzheimer's "

- **Lifestyle choices** are the greatest determining factor.
- **Stress reduction.** Cortisol is the stress hormone. Reduce your cortisol and you reduce your stress level thereby preserving brain cells.
- **Inflammation.** Inflammation in the body is the root cause of many complications, not the least of which is a contribution to dementia and Alzheimer's. Reduce your inflammation and reduce your chances of contracting Alzheimer's.
- **Sugars**, including high fructose corn syrup, have been found to be contributing factors to dementia and Alzheimer's.

Let's take each of these in detail one at a time.

Genetics

Alzheimer's and dementia may appear to run in your family. But, if your grandmother and your mother both lived with either of these conditions, this does not necessarily mean that genetics was the only factor. Research has identified common genes in AD patients however, there are other factors that create the conditions for the disease to take hold. For example, a person who possesses the common genes related to AD and who is also diabetic has an increased risk. Also, if there is a great deal of ongoing stress, which is an indication of elevated cortisol, the risk of AD is increased. As you continue reading, ask yourself if any of these factors apply to the people you have known who fell to Alzheimer's or dementia.

Lifestyle

As mentioned previously, there are multiple contributing factors, not the least of which is becoming sedentary with age.

It is of vital importance that we maintain strenuous physical activity throughout our years. Well-known fitness guru, Jack Lalane, maintained his exercise regimen until he passed from pneumonia at age 93. If you're not familiar with Jack's life and his protocols, I highly recommend a web search of his books and videos.

The benefits of regular, strenuous exercise are many. Those benefits relate directly to brain health in several ways. By maintaining healthy blood pressure and general heart health, our body is better equipped to feed our brains. Exercise also decreases stress and promotes mental focus.

The best way for seniors to ward off Alzheimer's disease may be to head to the gym and beeline for the weights.

The University of British Columbia released a new study on Tuesday linking strength training to better brain function.

Eighty-six older women, all already demonstrating early signs of dementia, were observed by researchers. Some took weight training courses, while others took aerobics and a third group did exercises for toning and balance.

After six months the group that lifted weights showed the biggest improvement in memory, attention span, problem-solving and decision-making.

Source: KPCC.org

A recent trial led by the University of Sydney in collaboration with the Centre for Healthy Brain Ageing at UNSW and the University of Adelaide found that increased muscle strength led to improved brain function in adults with Mild Cognitive Impairment (MCI).

Source: health times.com.au

More recent studies have found that lifting weights releases chemical compounds, such as serotonin, which improves mood, norepinephrine which boosts memory retrieval, BDNF or brain-derived neurotrophic factor which fosters long-term brain health and promotes new connections between brain cells, dopamine which is the motivation/reward chemical and endorphins which are the "feel good" chemicals, which also relieve fear and anxiety.

The benefits of regular, intense exercise at any age cannot be overstated. It's never too late to begin a weight training regimen. It is also never too early. If you've never partaken in a weight training program, there are thousands of YouTube videos that will help you to get started. Most gyms and fitness centers offer personal training and have specialized group programs for seniors at no additional cost. My recommendation for any senior is Anytime Fitness. I think of this franchise as the McDonalds of fitness. There are 2361 locations in the US, and they are in many countries worldwide. Members have 24-hour access and most locations offer a senior group program called "silver sneakers." If you are on Medicare in the US, your membership fees may be eligible to be paid for you. If you're retired and traveling, you'll find an Anytime Fitness location on your route.

You may also want to subscribe to a YouTube channel called "Athlean X" The instructor here is Jeff Cavalier. His channel is a comprehensive library of workouts for each body part, and you can find instruction that applies to beginners and up to the most advanced levels of fitness.

Cortisol

Numerous studies have linked stress and anxiety to Alzheimer's. Cortisol is the stress hormone. You may know someone with Alzheimer's who spent much of their life under stress. That person who overreacted to every situation, was depressed or was continually irritated, or was quick to anger. All of these behaviors indicate an elevated level of cortisol.

We've already discussed measures that can be taken to reduce stress and release your body's own healing chemicals to improve brain health but there is still more that can be done to reduce cortisol levels in the body by way of herbal supplementation.

As there is no exact science and science by any name is experimental, herbal remedies are no different. Some numerous herbs and roots have been found to lower cortisol levels, however, the exact dosages needed to make a significant change from one individual to the next will vary depending on nutrition, sleep, exercise regimen, and other factors. When starting an herbal remedy regimen, it's important to understand that you will need to start at a baseline and then adjust your dosage over time until you find the right dosage for you. I'll compile all of the information together in a chart towards the end.

Your beginning dosages should take into consideration your stage of treatment. If you're starting a preventive program before any symptoms appear, your dosage won't need to be the same as a person who has been diagnosed with the beginning stages of mild cognitive impairment. You may also have a reaction to certain herbs, such as nausea, which should pass within a few days. If reactions persist, there are alternatives to almost any herbal medication. Also, it must be taken into consideration that the body will only digest small doses of any nutrient and then discard any excess amounts consumed. For this reason, it is best to take small doses multiple times per day instead of a single dose per day.

You may consider different methods of consumption such as using herbs as a tea or to flavor foods. Ginger and turmeric, which we will discuss later, make a nice tea and can be drunk throughout the day and at night before bed. Both are also used as flavorings in many foods.

Let's take a look at herbal methods for reducing cortisol.

Chapter 3: Herbal Medications

Number 1
Ashwagandha

The use of Ashwagandha root in ancient medicine can be traced back to 6000 BC in India where it has long been known to relieve stress and anxiety and promote relaxation.

Here is a list of known benefits of Ashwagandha.
1. Reduces stress and anxiety.
2. Improves athletic performance.
3. Reduces symptoms of some mental conditions (i.e... bipolar disorder, depression, schizophrenia).
4. Increases testosterone.
5. Reduces blood sugar levels.
6. Reduces inflammation.
7. Improves brain function.
8. Improves sleep.

Number 2
Reishi Mushroom

This mushroom was discovered more than 2000 years ago by Chinese healers in The Changbai Mountains. Reishi has been found to support the immune and endocrine function as well as the endocrine system. In trials, has been proven to lower cortisol levels significantly. Ingestion is typically by capsule or hot tea.

(Side note: I've recently added Reishi to my regimen and found my mood to be significantly improved.)

Known benefits of Reishi include

- Boosts immune system
- Contains anti-cancer properties
- Fights fatigue and depression
- Decreases triglycerides
- Helps control blood pressure
- Detox liver
- Controls inflammation
- Improves respiratory health
- Improves cognitive function
- Boosts energy

Number 3.
Rhodiola Rosea

Multiple studies conclude that this flowering herb, grown in the high mountain regions of Europe and Asia acts as a balancing compound to maintain cortisol at normal levels. Buy in bulk to drink as a tea or in capsules.

Known benefits or Rhodiola Rosea;
1. Decreases stress
2. Fights fatigue
3. Reduces symptoms of depression
4. Improves brain function
5. Enhances exercise performance
6. Helps manage diabetes

Number 4;
Bacopa

An Indian herb that is also a stabilizing agent of cortisol. It has also shown benefits for improved cognition. Bacopa can be purchased as a powder, capsule, tea, or a syrup.

Known benefits of Bacopa
1. Contains powerful antioxidants
2. Reduces inflammation
3. Improves brain function

4. Reduces ADHD symptoms
5. Prevents anxiety and stress
6. Lowers Blood Pressure Levels
7. Fights certain cancers

Number 5;
L-Theanine

An amino acid found in black and green tea. In cases when you're avoiding caffeine, L- Theanine is still present in decaf or it can be purchased in capsules.

Known benefits of L-Theanine
1. Relieves stress and anxiety
2. Improves focus
3. Increases immune response
4. Decreases chances of ovarian and pancreatic cancer
5. Manages blood pressure
6. Lowers resting heart rate
7. Improves sleep

Some people find a side effect of Ashwagandha to be stomach upset. If you find this to be the case, my suggestion is to substitute with Reishi mushroom or one of the other possibilities on the list of Cortisol controlling remedies.

Chapter 4: Inflammation

Inflammation is a contributing factor or direct cause of numerous ailments including Alzheimer's, cancer, anxiety, depression, high blood pressure, stroke, heart disease, type 2 diabetes, allergies, asthma, skin diseases, arthritis, and many more. Reduce the inflammation and, chances are, your ailment goes away or at least stop causing problems for you.

Inflammation can occur anywhere in the body, including the brain. Inflammation in the brain can cause brain damage and lead to many serious conditions. Left unattended can become a contributing factor to Alzheimer's and dementia. In order for a treatment to achieve the intended goal, the remedy must be able to penetrate the blood-brain barrier.

The blood-brain barrier is a mesh of blood cells that protect the brain from most unwanted intruders. The BBB protects against pathogens while allowing passage of select nutrients such as glucose, fatty acids, and certain amino acids. This being the case, a remedy that lowers inflammation in the digestive tract may not work for the brain.

Let's look at remedies that lower inflammation while passing the blood-brain barrier.

Number 1
Ginger Root

Indigenous to China, the use of Ginger in traditional medicine can be traced back 5000 years.

Known benefits of Ginger root;
- Treats nausea
- Enhances a weight loss regimen
- Reduce symptoms of arthritis
- Lowers blood sugar
- Improves heart health
- Treats chronic indigestion
- Reduces menstrual pain
- Lowers cholesterol
- May prevent colon cancer
- Inhibits growth of infectious bacteria

Studies conducted by the Department of Pharmacognosy at Semmelweis University Budapest found that the rhizomes gingerol and shogaol, found in ginger root, were able to pass the BBB and perform its function as a treatment for inflammation as well as promote growth of new neurons.

Uses for ginger are too numerous to list. It can be used in baking, in a shaker as salt or pepper for any food, teas or as an additive for tea and coffee, pickled, or brewed to make beer or ginger ale. Although many micronutrients will be lost with the heat of cooking, the gingerols remain. For our purposes here, this is the goal. We want gingerols in the brain.

Number 2
Turmeric

The exact origin of turmeric is unknown but believed to be native to southern India and Indonesia. It has been used in medicine for thousands of years and is a member of the ginger family.

In India, where turmeric is widely used, turmeric is credited with Alzheimer's case numbers being 25% of the number of cases reported in The U.S. The active agent, curcumin, has been proven in multiple studies to maintain healthy blood sugar levels, aid in the burning of fat, and passes the blood-brain barrier to reduce inflammation and work to improve memory function. Like ginger, you will find that by using turmeric regularly, other ailments caused by inflammation will subside. Turmeric is used in baking as a spice and can be used to flavor coffee and tea. I carry a shaker with me at all times to sprinkle in coffee. Turmeric and ginger together brew nicely together as a tea. Both are also sold in capsule form.

Known benefits of Turmeric;
- Reduces inflammation
- Reduces chances of Alzheimer's
- Contains anti-cancer antioxidant compounds
- Boosts Brain Derived Neurotrophic Factor
- Lowers risk of heart disease

- Aids in the treatment of arthritis
- Treats depression
- Delay age-related disease

There is a remedy used in Chinese medicine for thousands of years, however, it has only become known and studied in the west over the past decade or so. I believe it warrants our attention as it relates to Alzheimer's and mild cognitive impairment and that is Lions Mane Mushroom.

I will refer you to an article that can be found at bebrainfit.com titled <u>HOW LION'S MANE MUSHROOM BENEFITS YOUR BRAIN.</u>

Clinical studies available are mostly animal studies and on small groups of human patients so results would be considered inconclusive. With that said, considering that side effects are minimal to none and preliminary tests showing improvement, there's no reason not to add this to your regimen.

Lions Mane can be purchased online in capsules or bulk and can be used as a tea or a spice.

Reported benefits of Lions Mane;
- Protects against Alzheimer's and dementia
- Relieves mild symptoms of depression and anxiety
- Speeds recovery of damaged nerves
- Protects against ulcers
- Reduces heart disease risk
- Aids in diabetes management
- Has been shown to kill certain cancer cells and slow the spread of cancer in animal studies
- Reduces inflammation and oxidative stress
- Improves immune system function

Research has found a link between the age-related decline of nitric oxide and AD as well as other diseases related to aging. Nitric Oxide or NO. NO is a vasodilator (widens blood vessels) that improves blood flow to every part of the body. NO becomes a gas in the blood, so it can pass the Blood Brain Barrier.

Many foods can be eaten that provide the necessary nutrients for your body to create NO, for example, beets, however, most of those foods contain sugars. This is where supplementation comes in. The amino acid, Citruline is named repeatedly in studies as a potent source of NO production. Citrulline can be purchased in capsules or flavored powder that can be mixed with water and actually tastes great.

Over the years, I have conducted many experiments using myself as the subject, by starting a supplement and then after a period of months or years stopping one particular supplement within my total regimen to see what the effect was. Most recently, I stopped taking citrulline malate for about two months and then I started back. I can tell you that this supplement has the greatest single effect on my performance and mood over any other that I've conducted this experiment with.

- Increases the size of blood vessels
- Lowers blood pressure
- Improves ED
- Increases blood flow
- Aids in the treatment of bipolar disorder
- Has shown signs of decreasing pain from sickle cell

While not directly related to brain function, there is a common household substance that aids in digestion which is important for overall health and ensures that nutrients do the job that our body requires. That is Apple Cider Vinegar. Your ACV should be organic and non-pasteurized. Two tablespoons in water are all that's needed to add needed digestive enzymes and balance your PH.

Although it may sound counterintuitive, ACV will reduce symptoms of acid reflux.

A solution of ACV before a meal and before pills or capsules will ensure proper digestion so your body receives the maximum benefit.

Chapter 5: Let's Talk About Sugar

The detriments of sugars in the diet are many. As we discussed previously, the causes and contributing factors linked to Alzheimer's are also many and a number of those can be traced back to low insulin. Insulin is the enzyme that makes blood cells receptive to glucose. Glucose is the energy source that is derived from sugars in the body. When we become insulin resistant, which is the case with a person who has Type 2 Diabetes, the brain is starved for energy.

In people without diabetes, 2 in 1000 will develop Alzheimer's while in people with Type 2 Diabetes the number balloons up to 6.25 in 1000. Many researchers focus their attention on the links between AD and diabetes. Alzheimer's is often referred to as Type 3 Diabetes.

You don't need to be diabetic to have negative effects from sugars. Research has found that non-diabetics with chronically elevated sugar levels are at greater risk for Alzheimer's.

Most people have felt something usually referred to as "brain fog." This is a result of too much sugar. The body's natural response of dumping insulin into your system to eat up the sugar causes you to have low sugar which cuts off your brain's energy supply.

So, what if there were another energy source for the brain? There is. It's called Ketones.

Ketones are triggered by a lack of glucose. When we lower our intake of sugars sufficiently, our liver produces ketones to supply our brain and the rest of the body with a cleaner, more efficient source of energy.

Ketones are produced in the liver from body fat in the absence of glucose(sugar). The body will always defer to sugars for energy first if sugars are present and then store whatever is leftover as fat in adipose tissue which is our fat storage container. Generally, after about 24 hours of fasting from sugars, your body will ease into a state of ketosis and begin using ketones as the primary source of energy. Another benefit to burning ketones as energy is the loss of body fat.

Now we need to identify sugar. When we think of sugar, most of us think of the white crystals that we have on the kitchen table. This is a processed and refined product of a plant. The fact is, sugar can be derived from virtually any plant.

We think of our daily glass of juice as healthy, not giving any thought to the amount of sugar that we're pouring into our digestive tract. Most foods are labeled with nutritive values, but labels can be misleading.

Most soft drink labels give you values based on a 12 Oz serving.

Home › Foods › Food List ›

Soda

Common Serving Sizes

1 can (12 fl oz) ▾

Calories	Fat	Carbs	Protein
140	0.04 g	36.05 g	0.26 g

There are 140 calories in 1 can of Soda.

Nutrition Facts

Serving Size	1 can (12 fl oz)

Amount Per Serving

Calories **140**

	% Daily Values*
Total Fat 0.04g	0%
Saturated Fat 0g	0%
Trans Fat -	
Polyunsaturated Fat 0g	
Monounsaturated Fat 0g	
Cholesterol 0mg	0%
Sodium 22mg	1%
Total Carbohydrate 36.05g	13%
Dietary Fiber 0g	0%
Sugars 33.76g	
Protein 0.26g	
Vitamin D -	
Calcium 4mg	0%
Iron 0.37mg	2%
Potassium 4mg	0%

🔒 fatsecret.com

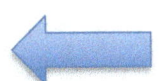

Note the serving size. This means the nutritional values are calculated for that amount NO MATTER THE BOTTLE OR PACKAGE SIZE. If the package size differs from the serving size, there will be a number indicating the number of servings per container or package.

Note the number of total carbohydrates in grams, then the total amount of sugar contained in the total number.
33.76 grams of sugar is more than you need in an entire day.

Orange and Apple juice labels often use a 1 Oz serving size to measure values. At equal servings, your favorite breakfast juice still gives you more than half of what you would ingest in a serving of soda.

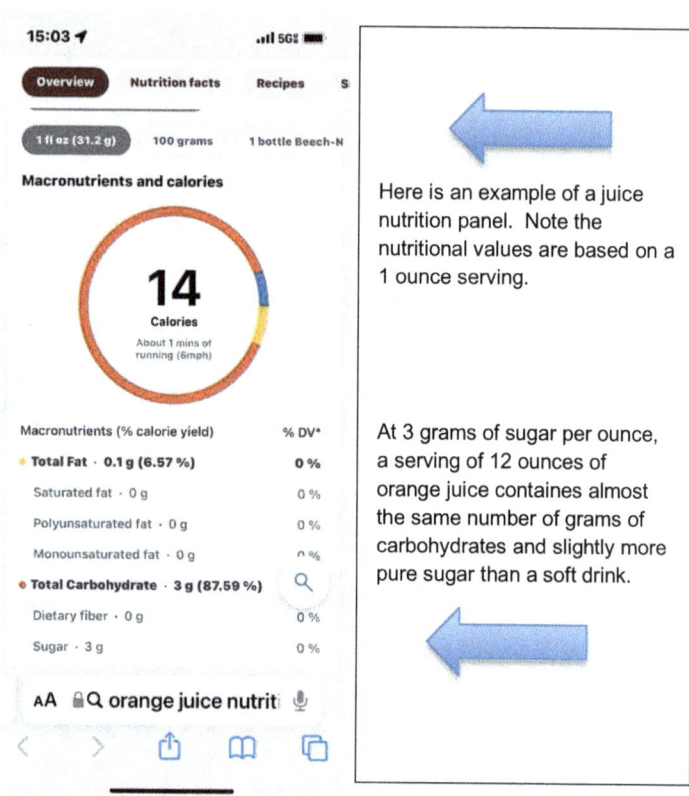

Here is an example of a juice nutrition panel. Note the nutritional values are based on a 1 ounce serving.

At 3 grams of sugar per ounce, a serving of 12 ounces of orange juice contains almost the same number of grams of carbohydrates and slightly more pure sugar than a soft drink.

Many foods you have been told are healthy should not be on your meal plan. For example, bananas are often recommended as a source of potassium and they are. However, the sugar content in bananas negates any benefit from other nutrients

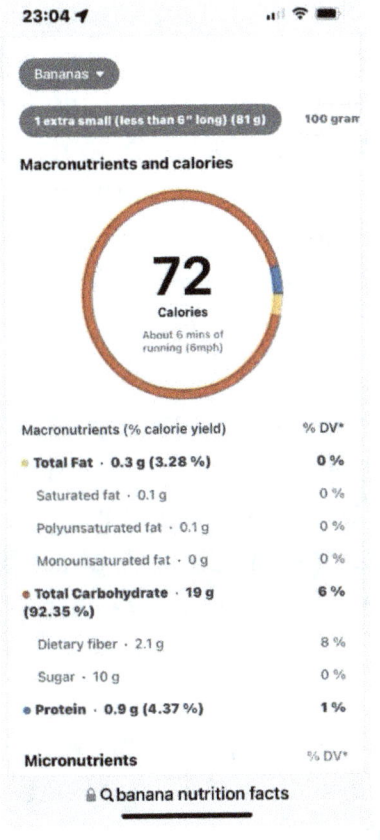

19 grams of carbs is 2/3 of your daily needs in one banana.

It's most important that you become a label reader. Measure portions and pay special attention to your carbohydrate intake. This number should be below 30 grams daily.

Following this protocol alone will make a significant change in your physiology in a short period. You will also begin to notice greater focus and mental clarity within days.

The idea of completely cutting sugars out of your life may be as foreign as moon dust to you. I've suggested this to many people over the years, often with the response, "Oh, I could never do that" or "I can't live without my chocolate candy." If this is your mindset, you must overcome it to win this war.

There are substitutes that you can adapt to. That is an important word, "adapt." To be a warrior in any fight, you must be prepared to adapt to change in the blink of an eye. Are you with me?

If you answered yes, then follow me through your kitchen. You may need to go to the grocery store when we're finished.

- Find all containers of **table sugar** and throw them in the trash.
- If you have **flour of any kind or corn meal**, sprinkle it in your backyard for the birds.
- **Bread,** including whole grain, cakes, pies, candy bars, and pastries go to the birds or the trash.
- Go into your pantry and take out **rice, potatoes, Pop Tarts, Rice Krispie treats, breakfast cereal, oatmeal, grits, cream of wheat, syrup, tomatoes, corn, yams, and any kind of noodles and take them to the food bank.**
- Now for the refrigerator; take out **fruits and fruit juices**, anything containing chocolate or a sweet flavoring or sugar like **coffee creamer**, or **margarine** (this doesn't include butter) throw in the trash, or pour liquids down the drain.

- If you have any **non-refrigerated fruits**, feed them to the birds and squirrels.
- Any **cooking oils or sprays except olive oil or coconut oil**, throw in the garbage.
- **Any nut** with exception of Brazil nuts, walnuts, and pecans, feed to your backyard pets. **Peanut butter in the trash**.

Now, let's create a shopping list;

Baking items
- Choose from one of these sweeteners; Splenda, stevia, or Truvia. Try them all, find your favorite, and adapt.
- Ginger root powder
- Turmeric powder
- Sea salt with iodine (if you don't have HBP)
- Black pepper
- Whey protein isolate or egg protein powder. (This can be found in most pharmacy aisles and will be used as a flour substitute.)
- Adobo seasoning

- Organic apple cider vinegar with mother. Braggs is the most common brand
- Olive oil and coconut oil. These should be your only cooking oils, but you may also use solid lard.

Veggies
- Avocados
- Celery
- Broccoli
- Organic Zucchini
- Cauliflower
- Brazil nuts
- Pecans
- Walnuts

Meats
- Fish
- Other seafood
- Bacon
- Sausage
- Ham
- Ground pork
- Steak
- Ground beef
- Chicken
- Turkey

Dairy

- Real cheese
- Sour cream
- Cream cheese
- Real butter without canola oil
- Whole cream
- Half and half
- Eggs

Drinks

- Coffee
- Black tea
- Green tea
- Ginger tea
- Bottled water

Nutrients are made up of 2 categories; macronutrients and micronutrients. Macronutrients are proteins, fats, and carbohydrates. Our bodies have a nutritional requirement for fats and proteins but not for carbohydrates. The Inuit Indians or Eskimo live thousands of years on fish, seal, caribou, and bear as vegetation doesn't grow in ice. You will need to keep count of your carbs and don't exceed 30 grams per day. Proteins should be about 40 grams per meal and eat fats until you're full. This may sound counterintuitive but, remember we're changing our fuel source from sugars to fats.

At this point, you may be thinking you'll never be able to eat in a restaurant again. This is not the case. I can order from the menu of almost any restaurant and maintain my regimen. It's usually as simple as having the waiter hold the side order. In most cases, the main course is meat and there are often a handful of veggies that you can eat such as broccoli with cheese or cauliflower with cheese. Be sure to sweeten your tea or coffee with the yellow sucralose sweetener or carry packets of Truvia or stevia with you to the restaurant. Ask for butter if they have real butter, sour cream, and cream cheese to add to whatever you're having. Once you've gone a few weeks into this regimen, you don't want a waiter to make the mistake of serving you tea sweetened with sugar.

Chaptr 7: OMAD

Eat to live, don't live to eat.

What is as important as what you eat
is how often you eat. We are a
gluttonous society. In the West, we've
become accustomed to plenty of
everything. We have bigger houses
with bigger closets full of more clothes,
bigger cars and more of them, and of
course, more food. We simply don't
need as much food as most of us eat.

The three-meal day began in the 17th
century when meals became more
ritualistic than nutritional. Eating
became part of weddings, meetings,
birthdays, and holiday celebrations,
and certain foods became designated
as the specific dish for the occasion.
Our ancestors before that time would
eat when they were hungry, without
regard for the time of day. At this point,
we are conditioned to be hungry in the
morning, at lunchtime, and in the early
evening. To heal ourselves, we must
recondition to our earlier physiological
requirements.

The acronym for One Meal A Day is becoming more popular among those who follow a ketogenic regimen. If you have never heard of this idea, you may be thinking that I've lost my mind and there's no way you'll be eating only one meal a day. Stick with me. I won't ask you to go cold turkey.

The road to OMAD doesn't happen in a day. Remember, I said we've been conditioned over the past 400 years to eat 3 times per day and we've been indoctrinated all of our lives by advertising that tells us that breakfast is the most important meal of the day and go to restaurant X for lunch and by this time your insulin is so dysregulated that you feel the urge to eat again before bed.

We begin with intermittent fasting. This protocol is being widely used in the Keto community and is adaptive in that you have a fasting period and then a feeding period with the feeding period becoming shortened over time until you only have one hour in the day in which you eat. Fasting is the fastest method to achieving a state of ketosis.

Many people start their intermittent fasting journey with a 16/8 protocol, which is fasting for 16 hours and then eating twice in eight hours. The recommendation is to skip breakfast and then have lunch from the prescribed menu around noon, then have dinner around 8 also from the prescribed menu.

How do we make it from 8 pm to noon the next day without eating? The answer is high fat.

Fats will stay in your stomach longer than proteins or carbohydrates which will carry you through the next morning. Do this for 30 days, then begin moving your lunch to a later time by one hour. By this time you will be adjusted to going without breakfast and moving lunch to a later time should be easier for you.

You are now at a 17/7 protocol. After 14 days, change your lunch again to one hour later. Now the protocol is 18 fasting hours and 6 feeding hours. Continue with this one-hour change every 14 days until you are only eating one time per day. You will begin to notice yourself becoming leaner. Your mood will change as you become more positive. Your mental focus improves. Cravings dissipate and over time will disappear.

You are now fully in a state of ketosis. One more step in this protocol. After 14 days, skip one day completely making for a 48-hour fast. Skip Sunday night until Monday night. This will ensure that you are fully keto and virtually all glucose is out of your system.

Chapter 8: The Herbal Regimen

Next, we lay the groundwork for your herbal, vitamin, and mineral protocol. We'll be adding a few things here that weren't previously mentioned as we've cut out some foods that contain these minerals, so we want to be certain that they are in sufficient supply. Your proteins will contain the necessary minerals however, we want to make sure our bases are covered.

We will be referring back to our earlier list of herbs to create a list of items that can be purchased online or at a vitamin store and then insert those into a daily regimen of:

- **A multivitamin that contains**
  - Zinc @ 50mg
  - Magnesium @ 50mg
  - B Vitamins 3,6&12 @ 1000 mcg each
  - Vitamin D3@ 15,000 IU
  - Selenium@ 50 mcg
  - Iodine@150mcg

- Boron @20mg
- Manganese @11mg
- Iron@45mg
- Calcium@2500
- Potassium@5000mg

- **Ashwagandha @300 mg**
- **A mushroom complex that contains Reishi and Lions Mane mushrooms @ 500 mg each**
- **Citrulline Malate powder @ 600 mg**

For those who are following this protocol for prevention, one time per day of each of these doses should be sufficient. Also, begin to make a practice of drinking coffee, and green and black tea as opposed to juice and soft drinks. With these drinks add ginger and turmeric powder. You can also purchase ginger root and make a tea by chopping the root and then boiling it until the water becomes light brown. The liquid can be sweetened to your preference and then you may want to try sweetening the root after it's boiled and then eat it as a snack.

Always precede vitamins and food with 2 teaspoons of apple cider vinegar. This can be mixed with water and will help with digestion. Also, drink a ginger and turmeric tea before bed. This will help maintain insulin levels while you sleep.

If you have already begun to experience signs that give you a reason to be concerned, you should increase the frequency of your dosages remembering that taking a larger dose at once is not useful as your body will only use a small amount of any nutrient, regardless of the size of the dose. This being the case, refer to the chart below.

	Morning	Afternoon
Citrulline Malate	600mg	
Multi Vitamin	as directed On bottle	
Ashwagandha	300 mg	300 mg

Reishi and lion's mane mushroom	500 mg Each	500 mg Each
Ginger tea	1 cup	1 cup
Coffee or green tea with turmeric	throughout the day	throughout the day

Remember to mix a solution of 2 tablespoons of Apple cider vinegar in water before supplements and food.

You may have been already diagnosed. At this point, you're fighting for life. Now is the time to saturate your body and brain with these compounds and go all in on Keto and exercise.

We increase the dosages to four per day of most of the supplements as follows;

	9 am	1 pm	5 pm	9 pm

Citrulline Malate	600 mg			
Ashwagandha	300mg	300 mg	300 mg	300 mg
Reishi/ Lions Mane	500 mg	500 mg	500 mg	500 mg
Ginger Tea	1 cup	1 cup	1 cup	1 cup
Coffee or green tea with turmeric	all day	all day	all day	all day
multivitamin	as directed			

Chapter 9: Exercise

There are a few things to consider before starting your exercise regimen.

If you've never undertaken an exercise regimen or if you have already been diagnosed with high blood pressure or heart disease, or if you are overweight, you need to work on your heart strength first. Keep in mind that this will be a process to get you to a weight-lifting regimen and you will need a strong heart to get there.

You will need a heart rate meter. Most cardiovascular equipment today will have a meter onboard or you can download an app that monitors your heart rate onto your phone. Begin with the treadmill. Walk slowly as you monitor your heart rate. Your rate should reach 120 beats per minute. The immediate goal is to build your stamina until you can sustain this rate for 30 minutes. Reaching this goal may take two weeks or two months. Don't allow yourself to be discouraged by slow progress. You didn't get to your current physical state overnight so you won't get to where you need to be overnight. Remember, this is a fight for your life.

Once you've achieved the first goal, it's time to move on to another stage of the fitness regimen. At this point, you may need to purchase time with a personal trainer in order to learn how to use the machines. If hiring a trainer is a financial burden, you can look for videos on YouTube. All that is necessary to find a video on the how-to of a particular piece of weight-lifting equipment is to read the name on the side of the machine. If you don't see it, ask someone what it is and then open your YouTube app and type in "how to use a leg extension machine" or "how to use a shoulder press machine." You may also need to include the brand name of the machine in your search as there are some differences between brands.

You're going to experience soreness but don't allow this to be a deterrent. As your soreness goes away, you're starting to experience benefits; your immune system comes alive, endorphins begin to respond and you will feel the release of hormones that you haven't experienced for years. After some time, you will experience an almost narcotic dopamine response. This is the point at which exercise has become like an addiction and you feel drawn to the gym. For a period of time, you'll be operating on pure willpower. Keep motivating yourself even when you don't feel like going. After some weeks or months, working out will be something you can't wait to do.

Chapter 10: Take Your Brain To The Gym!

Now that we have your body on the right track and you're feeding your brain with high-quality nutrients, we need a workout regimen for your brain.

There have been numerous studies just in the past decade that indicate that multi-lingual people are many times less likely to have AD or dementia. One such study conducted by researchers at The University of Waterloo, examined 325 Nuns who were from The Sisters Of Notre Dame of The US. They found that of the sisters who spoke 4 or more languages, only 6% developed dementia compared to 31% for those who only spoke 1 language.

It's never too late to begin a language learning program. Numerous free apps can be downloaded to your phone and offer a broad selection of language choices. My personal choice is Duolingo which is where I study Spanish, Portuguese, and Japanese. This app will start you at the very basic level and bring you to the conversational.

Begin with a language that shares characters with your native language, for example, if you're a native English speaker, you might choose Spanish, French, or German. After you feel comfortable with the app and you've established a routine, choose a language with different characters, such as Japanese or Russian. Make a practice of exercising your language skills every time you go to the restroom, sit in a waiting room, before you watch TV, or during a commercial.

As you become more familiar with your new language, consider searching for meet-up groups that regularly gather to practice in social settings. You can find these groups on sites like meetup.com and Craigslist.org.

Chapter 11: Hygiene Products

Many of the hygiene products we use are loaded with chemicals, namely aluminum compounds, which have been found in the brains of AD patients, and propylene glycol which blocks nutrients in the small intestine, preventing them from feeding your brain and the rest of your body. This includes deodorant, toothpaste, shampoo, soap, and lotion.

Avoid products containing
- Aluminum
- Parabens
- Propylene glycol

There are natural alternatives for all of these products.

Natural deodorants
- Ursa Major
- Real Purity
- Piper Wai
- Dove 0% Aluminum
- Native
- Routine Superstar
- Every Man Jack.

Natural Soaps

- Caswellmassey.com has soaps, shaving creams, lotions, and fragrances for men and women.
- Rockymountainsoap.com has a complete line of personal care products.
- Mistral classic bar soap
- Glossier Body exfoliating soap
- Yes to coconut hydrating milk bar soap
- Every Man Jack

Natural toothpaste

- Baking soda
- Hydrogen peroxide

Natural lotions

- Williams-Sonoma.com
- Skin food body butter
- Sephora
- Briogeo

- Burt's Bees Milk and Honey
- Follain

You can find these on individual company websites or on Amazon and eBay. Palmers and Burt's Bees are available at any major pharmacy. Every Man Jack products are also available at Pilot Truck Stops. I know, weird.

Bisphenol-A is an industrial chemical used in many plastic products. It can be found in food containers, baby bottles, plastic water bottles, and hygiene products. You may have noticed some manufacturers have begun adding a "BPA Free" stamp to their products since the discovery of BPA hazards.

Research has found that BPA exposure is so widespread that most people over the age of 6 have a measurable amount in their urine. BPA mimics the hormone estrogen so binding to estrogen receptors and influencing bodily processes such as growth, cell repair, energy levels, and reproduction. It has also been found to impair communication between neuro processers in the brain.

When purchasing plastic storage bags or containers, look for the BPA Free label. Also, look for foods packaged in glass or metal containers. Most bottled water is packaged in plastic bottles, however, many bottlers have made the change to BPA-free bottles. A list of those is below.

- Fiji
- Evian
- Dasani
- Essential
- Just water
- Core hydration
- Perrier
- Lifewtr
- Propel
- Nestle Pure
- Waiakia Hawaiian
- Voss Artesian
- Glaceu smart
- Aquafina
- Icelandic

- Poland springs
- Perfect hydration
- Ice mountain
- Acqua Panna
- Penta

Fortunately, many of the protocols in this guide will aid in the expedient removal of residual BPAs that may be lingering in your system. Sweat is the most effective flushing mechanism.

Fluoride is found in most public water systems and is a poison. Sodium fluoride occurs in nature and can be found in well water and other natural sources, however, it shouldn't be confused with the man-made chemical fluoride. It is a compound that is used in rat poison yet fluoride is used in virtually every public water system in the developed world. Regulatory bodies claim that such a small amount is added to our water that it is harmless, however, these entities don't account for fluoride buildup in the pineal gland and thyroid gland as well as the weakening of your bones due to fluorosis.

The pineal gland is a small endocrine gland that sits near the middle of your brain at the top of the vertebrae. Its function is to regulate the circadian rhythm by secreting melatonin. Fluoride attacks the pineal gland and reduces the excretion of melatonin, which is why we have trouble sleeping as we age. It is also a pro-oxidant. Oxidation in the body, particularly the brain, creates numerous malfunctions which is why anti-oxidant foods and supplements are widely recommended, both by herbalists and medical scientists.

The thyroid is an endocrine gland that regulates metabolism. Research has found that thyroid dysfunction has been linked to reversible cognitive impairment. A thyroid test is part of the lab screening for AD.

It's virtually impossible to completely eliminate fluoride from your life as it is in the water we use for cooking and bathing as well as toothpaste and other hygiene products. The good news is that we can flush the neurotoxin from the thyroid and pineal gland. In following the protocols in this guide you are already flushing the fluoride by ingesting turmeric and the trace mineral Boron which you should have in your multivitamin. There is an additional herbal source that, according to The Indian Council of Medical Research, will expedite the excretion of fluoride from bones as well as the pineal and thyroid and that is Tamarind Leaves. Tamarind can be found online and in herb shops. the leaves can be eaten raw or can be used to make tea. Use this remedy as a boost instead of a part of your daily regimen as you already have two compounds working in your favor to eliminate the toxin. Take one day each month to drink Tamarind tea several times that day.

Chapter 12: Commercial Farming and Toxic Chemicals

Most of us don't give much thought to the origin of our food, we just make the trip to the grocery store and buy what we need. We trust that our system of oversight has taken care of all of the necessary safety guidelines to ensure compliance of all who are involved in the supply chain at every point. We believe without question that if any toxin happens to make it into our food source, it will be quickly detected and eliminated. Recalls happen frequently so the regulatory process is working, right?

It is likely that if I walk into your basement, you have a bottle of the weed killer RoundUp. This herbicide is also used in commercial farming to kill weeds that are grown near crops like corn, soy, almonds, sugar beets, and many more foods. The target food plants have been genetically modified to resist the chosen herbicide so that the only plants killed are the weeds. This creates less work for the farmer, however, has several other less favorable effects.

The active ingredient in RoundUp is Glyphosate which received FDA approval for commercial use in 1974. Glyphosate works by inhibiting the production of a plant enzyme that plays a role in the synthesis of three amino acids named phenylalanine, tyrosine, and tryptophan. RoundUp is applied to the leaves and then spreads throughout the plant, preventing the formation of these proteins. Although the intended crop that has been genetically modified is not killed, the amino acids in the plant are still blocked therefore, when those plants are eaten they do not contain some of the amino acids that are necessary for our nutrition. Glyphosate also binds to metals, which are the minerals in soil that feed the plants and prevents the minerals from being used by the plant, thereby depriving the plant and the food consumer – human and livestock --of the nutritional benefits that the plant would otherwise provide.

Here are a few things that I would like to point out with regard to soil. everything that our body requires to be properly nourished begins in the soil. Since the beginning of time, nutrients have been returned to the soil through weeds, worms, insects, fungi, and bacteria. all of the nutrients begin here and are then taken into the plants that either we or livestock eat. Traditionally, farmers would begin their season by tilling soil that was covered in weeds, the weeds would go into the soil and except for the seeds, would die and compost, giving the soil the nutrients needed for the plant and us. In addition, worms would dig through the soil, leaving nitrates behind, further fortifying the soil. Also, as the soil naturally retains moisture, bacteria and fungus would form, eventually becoming part of the digestive enzymes that we need in our gut. All of these are killed off by glyphosate, making the soil weak and creating an additional need for chemical fertilizers to feed the plants which are not being fed by the soil, adding unnatural and potentially toxic chemicals to our bodies.

The unused portions of glyphosate and other chemicals go into the soil and air and eventually make their way into the water table. Although, it's virtually impossible to completely avoid glyphosate, we can and should reduce our intake and take measures to eliminate this toxic chemical from our bodies.

Step 1. Most of the foods I listed here have already been placed on the do not eat list, however, to illustrate the widespread use of glyphosate, I will add them to this list of foods to avoid also. Any foods found on this list that are also on the DO EAT list should be purchased from organic sources.

- Corn
- Soybeans
- Rapeseed/canola
- Potato
- Papaya
- Zucchini/squash
- Beet/sugar Beet
- Alfalfa
- Flax

- Apple
- Plum
- Farm raised salmon
- Cloned meat
- Yeast
- Pineapple
- Rice
- Sugarcane
- Tomatoes
- Wheat
- Chickory
- Melons(all varieties)
- Banana

You can find more detail on each of these at organichawaii.org

Step 2. You are already taking some measures to speed the elimination process, however, a daily dose of activated charcoal will remove glyphosate and other chemicals as they are introduced into your system.

Refer to these articles for more on glyphosates possible health risks. Verywellhealth.com (does glyphosate cause cancer?)

Also

Food.Berkeley.edu

(Childhood Exposure to Common Herbicide May Increase the Risk of Disease in Young Adulthood)

Beginning The Journey

If you have decided to join me in this war of Alzheimer's the time to start is now. I have included a few Keto recipes on the following pages to get you startedand I will be offering additional resources in my Facebook group, Brain Health Protocol.

I would like to stay in touch with readers of this guide. If you have questions, comments, or stories to share, please email me at brainhealthprotocol@gmail.com

Recipes

Here are a few recipes to get you started.

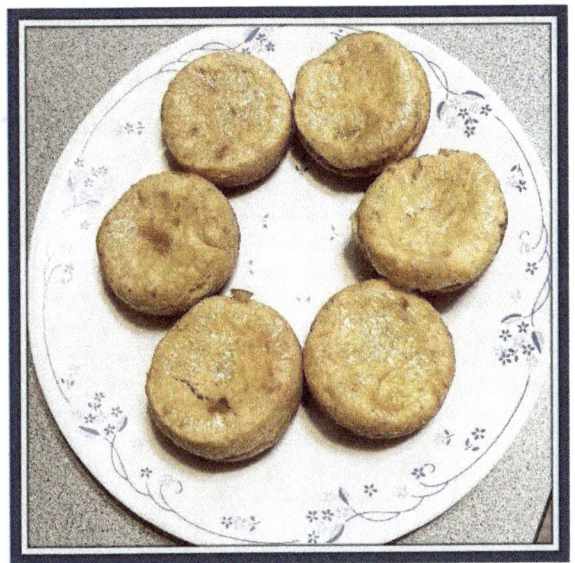

Keto Muffins
Ingredients

3 eggs
1 8oz package of cream cheese
1 cup of Splenda or other sucralose
sweetener
1 tsp of your favorite flavoring (vanilla,
almond, etc.)
8 scoops of whey protein isolate
3 tsp water
½ cup Brazil nuts, pecans or walnuts

- Preheat oven to 350.
- Grind nuts into a powder in food processor.
- Mix all other ingredients into a creamy batter then add nuts.
- Pour into a non-stick muffin pan or line with muffin pan liners.
- Bake for 25 minutes or until golden brown on top.
- This will make 12 muffins

Recipe courtesy of Jean Sargent

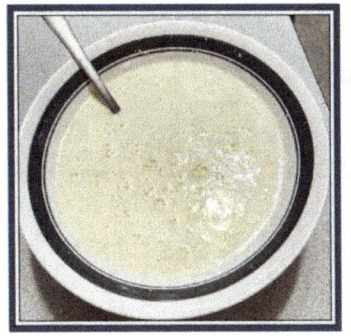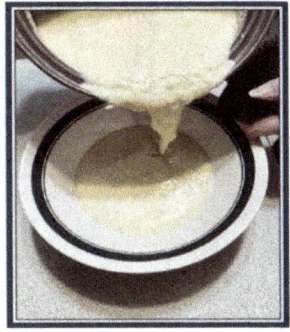

Cream of Celery Soup

Ingredients

1 stalk fresh celery
⅓ cup whipping cream
⅓ cup half and half
⅓ cup your favorite grated cheese
Sea salt to your taste

- Wash celery, chop into 1 inch pieces. Simmer in enough water to cover until soft, about 10 minutes. Drain then grind in blender or food processor until almost smooth.....
- Mix ingredients together in a pan and bring to a simmer for about 5 minutes, just until all ingredients are hot. DO NOT BOIL. CREAM WILL SCORCH EASILY.

Recipe courtesy of Jean Sargent

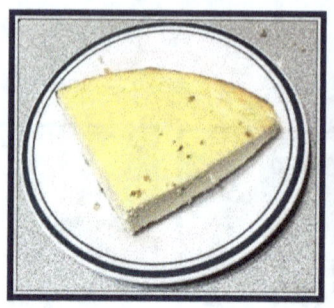 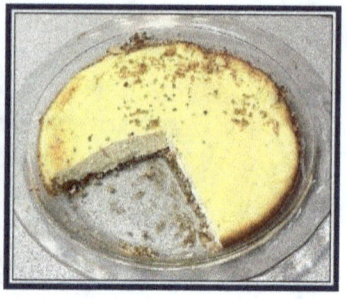

Keto Cheesecake

Ingredients

3 8 ounce packages of cream cheese
3 eggs
1 cup Splenda
1 tsp your favorite flavoring
½ cup Brazil nuts, walnuts or pecans
2 or 3 tablespoons olive oil as needed

- Preheat oven to 350°
- In food processer or blender, grind nuts until they are fine.
- Mix ground nuts with enough olive oil to hold the mixture together.
- Press nut mixture into a 9 inch pie plate across the bottom and up the sides. You can use another pie plate to compress the mixture and make it solid.
- Place unboxed cream cheese in microwave safe bowl. Microwave for 30 second intervals until soft enough to mix. DO NOT GET THE CREAM CHEESE HOT.

Microwave just long enough to soften. Alternatively, leave the cream cheese on the counter for an hour before starting.

- Combine cream cheese, Splenda, eggs and flavoring in mixer and whip until smooth. Do not overmix. Pour into lined pie pan.
- Bake 30 minutes
- Allow to cool before slicing.

Recipe courtesy of Jean Sargent

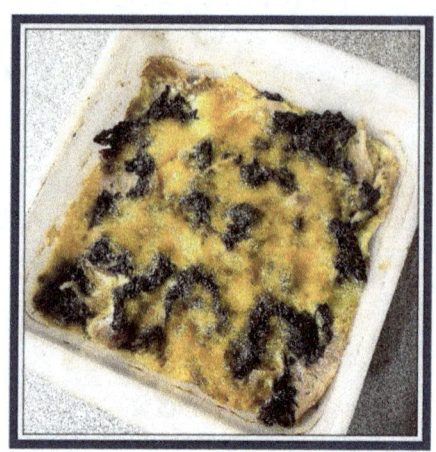

Keto Cauliflower/Pork Casserole

Ingredients

1 small pack of frozen cauliflower (usually 10 02 12 ounces) or similar amount of fresh
1 cup your favorite grated cheese
½ lb ground pork
2 tsp Rosemary
1 tsp mayonnaise
Salt to your taste

- Preheat oven to 350.
- Boil cauliflower in water until soft, then drain.
- Mix ground pork with rosemary, salt, mayonnaise.

- Coat 8 or 9 inch baking dish with olive oil then layer bottom of dish with half the cheese.
- Layer pork and cauliflower into dish then top with remainder of cheese.
- Bake for 45 minutes at 350.

Recipe courtesy of Jean Sargent

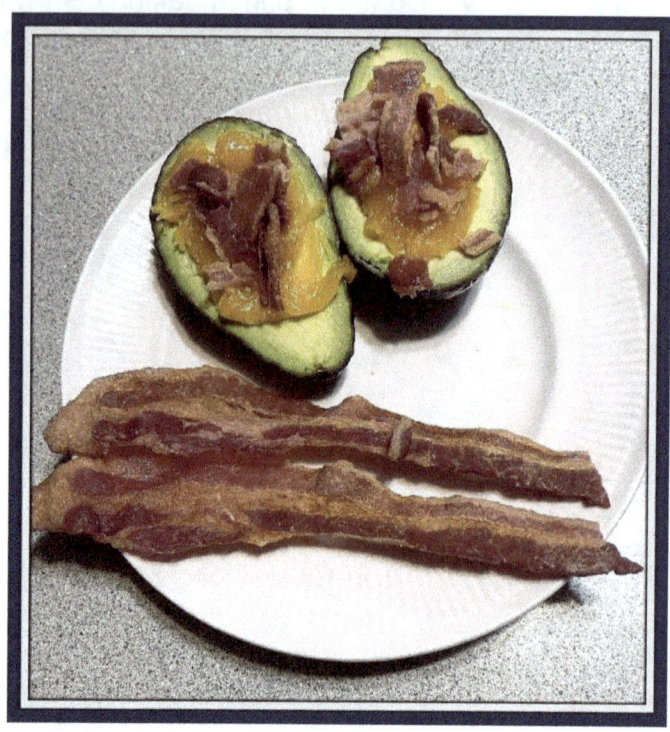

Avocado, Cheddar, and Bacon.

This is not so much a recipe so much as just directions for a quick low carb snack or meal. This one would be great for the first meal during your intermittent fasting transition to One Meal a Day.

- Cook bacon in the microwave for crispy, crunchy strips.

- On a microwave safe plate, melt some grated cheese just until it is soft. Depending on your microwave, this usually takes 30 seconds or so.

- Wash and halve an avocado, remove the seed.

- With a spatula place the cheese on the avocado as shown. Crumble the bacon on top.

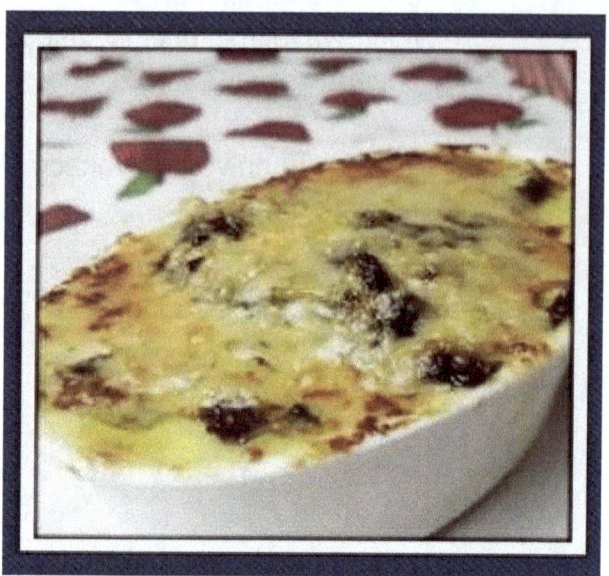

Three Cheese Creamed Spinach

Ingredients

3 Bags (8 ounces Each) Fresh Spinach
1 Large Onion
1 Cup Heavy Cream
4 Ounces Grated Cheddar
8 Ounces Provolone
3 Ounces Grated Parmesan
3 Tablespoons Butter
1/2 Teaspoon Minced Garlic (Or 1 to 2
Cloves)
Salt and Pepper to Taste.

NOTE: This will be cooked under the broiler in your oven. Before starting, lower your oven rack one position so that the flame from the broiler won't scorch your cheese.

- In a deep 10 inch skillet or Dutch oven, melt butter on low heat.
- Slice onion in half from top to bottom, then slice each half into ½ inch slices.
- On medium low heat, sauté onion slices in butter until they become translucent and start to show some browning.
- Add garlic.
- Add the raw spinach in batches by filling your pan as much as you can, sprinkling a little salt on top, cover for3 minutes and allow it to wilt, then repeat until all the spinach is in the pan. This usually takes 3 batches in a skillet. If you are using a Dutch oven, you may be able to do it in one batch.
- After all the spinach has wilted, spoon off about half the liquid.
- Add heavy cream.
- Add provolone cheese and allow it to melt.
- Add cheddar cheese and allow it to melt.

- Spoon the mixture into 4 individual 8 ounce ramekins or baking dishes OR into 1 8 or 9 inch casserole dish.
- Cover the top with the grated parmesan.
- Place in oven under the broiler for about 4 minutes

Recipe courtesy of Debbie's Back Porch. Video at https://youtu.be/deZHn0iBkqw

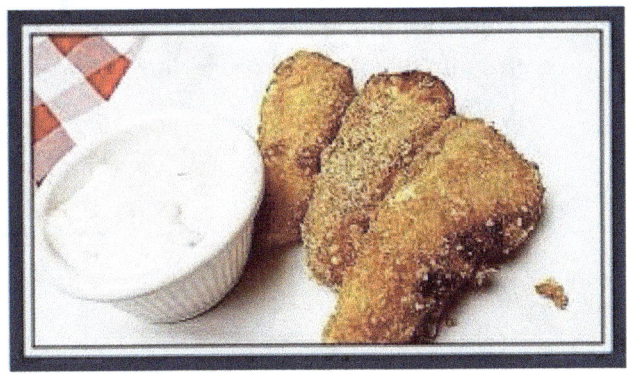

Crunchy Cheese Wedges

Ingredients

1/2 Pound Queso Fresco. NOTE; You want to use a fresh cheese that does not melt easily.
2 to 3 Ounces of Pork Rinds
1 Egg
1 Teaspoon Water
Oil for Frying (coconut or olive oil)

Grind pork rinds in food processor into a coarse meal, the texture of corn meal.
Beat the egg and water in a bowl.
Cut cheese into 1.2 inch wedges as pictured.
Dip each cheese wedge into the egg wash, then the pork rinds making coating as solid as possible.
Heat oil to medium heat in cast iron or non-stick skillet.

Carefully place wedges in hot oil for one minute, turn. Cook an additional one minute.

Drain on paper towel then serve hot.

Recipe courtesy of Debbie's Back Porch. Video athttps://youtu.be/vyCAmWgvX9Q

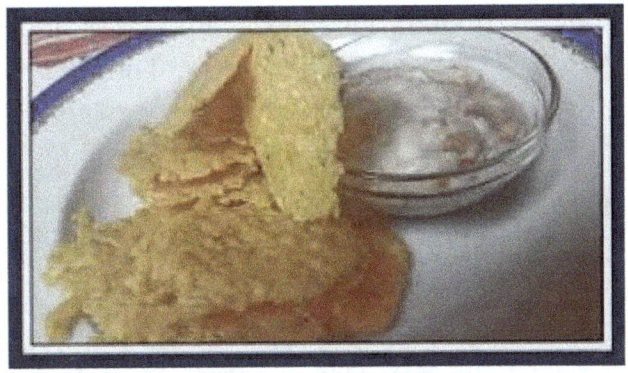

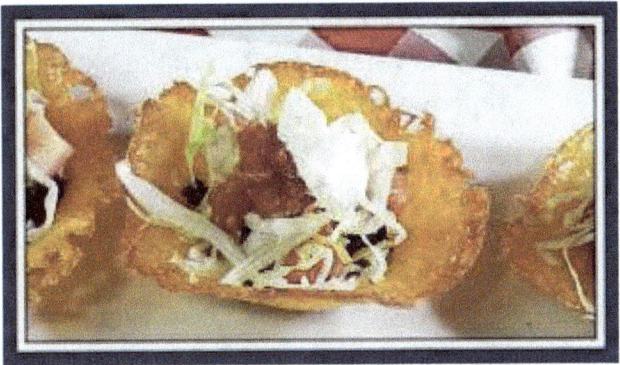

Cheese Crisps

Cheese crisps are a perfect keto snack, but they are super expensive. Luckily they are easy and quick to make. This is not really a recipe, just directions. These can be made as small chips, or larger to shape as taco shells. salad bowls or tostado flats.

Choose your cheese. Freshly grated parmesan works well, but I have used cheddar, asiago, gruyere , and jack. Pre-grated cheese is fine, but the texture is a little different. Pre-grated cheese gets a bad rap because there is a small amount of cellulose added for texture, but cellulose is not a bad thingm so use it if you want. I like the finely grated Mexican blend product and it gives me good results when I want to make a shaped finished product like bowls or shells.

Preheat oven to 350.
Line a cookie sheet with parchment paper or a silicone liner.

Make piles of the grated cheese on the paper/liner and gently pat them down into your desired size. They should be about 1/8 inch thick. Not solid, but compact. You want some little air pockets

The amount of cheese depends on the finished size you want. Chips should be about 1 ½ inches. Tacos and bowls 3 to 4 inches. Play with it until you get the size you want. Be sure to allow enough space between each chip to allow for melting.

Bake for 15 minutes for chips. Larger pieces may need up to 20 minutes. Check after 12 minutes to make sure they don't scorch. Ovens vary.

When they are fully melted, transfer chips to a paper towel to drain. Larger pieces can be molded over a small bowl or the end of a cup or drinking glass. Taco shells can be draped over the rim of a large bowl or pan to shape the fold.

Allow them to fully cool before using. Chips can be bagged for later use after they are fully cooled, but they are not for long term storage and should be consumed within 24 hours.

Recipe courtesy of Debbie's Back Porch. Videos at https://youtu.be/bhG4ihWfKs8 and https://youtu.be/sVISEWacOak

www.ingramcontent.com/pod-product-compliance
Lightning Source LLC
Chambersburg PA
CBHW070748220526
45467CB00018B/1488